Emergency Preparedness Plan

A Workbook for Caregivers, People with Disabilities,
the Elderly and Others

By Laura George, Emergency Management Disability Liaison

Contributing Author Jackie Schwabe, CEO, MindLight, LLC

Copyright © 2015, 2019 Laura George

Published by Vacano Creative
2350 NE 134th Place
Portland, OR 97230

Cover illustration by Charlotte George

Cover design by Vacano Creative

Layout by Vacano Creative

Contributing Author Jackie Schwabe

ISBN:9586567X

ISBN-13:   978-1795865678

Dedication

Spike was my husband of 27 years, in addition to being father and friend to all who knew him. He passed away after spending the last six years of his life with a spinal cord injury and three rare life threatening neurological disorders. Only five months after the spinal cord injury while I was pregnant, we found ourselves facing a hurricane head-on. Having no idea on how to become emergency prepared to address disabilities and disasters we realized we would have to decide between his life with a newly diagnosed disability and the life of our unborn child. Addressing a disability, a pregnancy and a disaster at the same time woke us up to the importance of being emergency prepared.

This book is dedicated to him, because if it was not for the experience, we would never have known of the need for education and awareness on the topic.

For Spike, because everyone's life is sacred!

(Thank you, Charlotte, for drawing the picture!)

Table of Contents

Introduction

Over a decade ago I learned the hard way that there was no education upon discharge from a hospital with a new disability as to how to prepare for the hurricane season. My husband and I came up with a document shortly after and brought it to his subsequent hospital visits. The medical staff would distribute them within two hours and always ask for more. As his health worsened and became more complicated, we realized it would be good to have the data easily accessible for our piece of mind and as an informative tool in terms of time response for the first responders we worked with.

That idea has now grown into a book which is designed to be a tool to empower caregivers, persons with disabilities, the elderly and others to be in control and knowledgeable when encountering emergency situations. When worked on as a collaborative community effort it will serve as a tool to help aid the first responder in giving care more quickly and efficiently. We worked together with the community to help form positive collaborations between carees, caregivers, and first responders.

It has been intentionally designed to *not* be specific to one type of disability since most people will need to fill out information that crosses over several disabilities.

As much as possible, size 14-point font was used instead of the traditional 10 or 12 to help give relief from reading tiny print. Very few directions were entered in on each page, so it would be easy to understand what information needed to be circled or written in.

It is not expected that this workbook will be completed overnight or even address all concerns. Rather, its purpose is to provoke thought, discussion and education around all items related to emergencies (weather, medical, etc.). The end result of this is to aid you in emergency and chaotic times when we tend to be overwhelmed in stressful situations with volumes of details to remember and that requires instant decision making.

I warmly invite you to think of this as your first responder brain in an emergency!

Definitions

In order to better understand the point of view of each topic requiring inputted information, you may want to become familiar with the following terms.

You may also want to add in local acronyms and terms to refer back to.

Caree - Person with the disability who needs assistance with a daily living activity or activities.

Caregiver - Family member, Friend or Partner who gives care and assists the caree with any daily living activities that they may not be able to perform by themselves. They may be not paid or paid.

Caretaker - Generally a person that works at a cemetery taking care of the deceased but is sometimes used to refer to someone that is helping a non-family member in times of crisis.

PCA (Personal Care Assistant) – Generally, thought of as a paid employee/caregiver to help the caree with daily living activities.

Editing Update

Use this page to register every time you make a change to the book. Keeping a record of updates allows those referring to the book to know how current the information is.

Date	Change Made	Who Entered Change

Basic Information

Don't panic! Instead write it down so you have less to remember during an emergency!

Name:	
Date of Birth:	Social Security Number:
Contacts: Yes No	Glasses: Yes No
Address:	
City, State, Zip, County:	
Email:	
Phone:	Cell:
Health Insurance: Company Name: Phone: Plan #: Group:	Company Name: Phone: Plan #: Group:

Home Details/Connections

This is basic household information that is easily forgotten until accessibility has been lost. Knowing at least the name of the utility company can be helpful to getting the power back on.

<table>
<tr>
<td>Utility Companies

Don't make the call where the gas is leaking. Get a safe distance away from the leak so a spark doesn't cause a fire!</td>
<td>(Include Name, Phone #, Account # & Password if Applicable)

Electrical:

Gas:

Water:

Who can turn these on/off?</td>
</tr>
<tr>
<td colspan="2">On Life Dependent Equipment? Yes   No
Equipment Provider Name:
Equipment Provide Contact Information:

If yes, is it Oxygen or _______________________________________
I use it to/for:
If yes, is it Dialysis or _____________________________________
Dialysis Center Name:
Dialysis Center Contact Information:
Receive transfusions (days/week):
Received extra transfusion before upcoming disaster? Yes   No</td>
</tr>
<tr>
<td>Connected to community Code Red or Smart911 service?</td>
<td>Yes   No</td>
</tr>
<tr>
<td>Pre-registered with local disaster/shelter program?</td>
<td>Yes   No</td>
</tr>
<tr>
<td>Do you have a Weather Alert Radio?</td>
<td>Yes   No</td>
</tr>
<tr>
<td>>>> Is adaptive equipment required to hear/see it?
If yes, contact:</td>
<td>Yes   No</td>
</tr>
<tr>
<td>Home/Rental Insurance:
Policy Number: Phone:</td>
<td>Yes   No</td>
</tr>
</table>

Take a local Community Emergency Response Team (CERT) or Red Cross class to learn more. (This does not mean that you *have to* continue working with them after taking the class, but they will welcome your time and input.

Communication

<table>
<tr><td>

My First Language is:

English   Spanish   Russian   French

Other:

</td></tr>
<tr><td>

I use technology to communicate. Yes   No

What is important to know about how I can communicate:

</td></tr>
<tr><td>

I am: Deaf   Hard of Hearing   Deaf/Blind   Blind/Low Vision

I use: Technology   American Sign Language (ASL)   Lip Reading

        Communication Access Relay Technology (CART)   Caption

I need: Large Print   Braille

I need assistance with writing: Yes   No

I need assistance with:

</td></tr>
<tr><td>

Other:

</td></tr>
</table>

Calling 911: Operators will look for the *COT*

If you ever find yourself in a position of having to call 911 for assistance here are some notes to make the call more productive in helping your caree and the 911 operator address the situation even more quickly.

CALM
*   Make sure that your caree is in a safe state or location
*   Take a moment to close your eyes and breath slowly once or twice.
*   Have someone nearby make the call for you or take over while you make the call.

ORGANIZE
*   Know the complete location address and main cross roads.
*   Phone number you are calling from & an alternate in case the battery dies or a number is misdialed.
*   Collected short thoughts about the emergency, and details.
    *   *Ex: Daily Diagnosis (Paralysis, Autism, MRSA, Heart Condition)
    *   *Ex: Medication (XX mgs @ 2/day of antibiotic to treat -condition-)
    *   *Ex: Physical status: (Not breathing for X mins., blood pressure is 200/300, body is bleeding profusely, right eye is not lined up properly)

TALK
*   Call the 911 Operator and speak calmly identifying that you have an emergency.
*   Answer their questions in the order they ask them.
    *   *Location and Phone Number
    *   *Short specific details about the emergency
    *   *Follow the operator's instructions and ask any last questions.
    *   *Do not end the call "until" instructed to do so!

** (If you live in a uniquely drawn city/county jurisdiction, you may need to identify first that the operator has to transfer you to a different 911 jurisdiction.)

Additional notes:
If your caree has paralysis, you want to pre-identify to make sure that there is enough manpower to lift them. You also want to say "ambulance with transport" which means that it comes with a gurney to accommodate the person who cannot walk.

It also helps to pre-identify if the caree's first language is other than English, is Deaf/Hard of Hearing, has Vision challenges or any other disability or condition that might require additional technical training or knowledge by the arriving first responders.

See also www.911.gov.

Unique Considerations

<table>
<tr><td colspan="2">Primary Diagnosis is:
Impact is: (Exp. Diabetes causes foot pain.)</td></tr>
<tr><td colspan="2">Challenges Are:</td></tr>
<tr>
<td>

Mobility:

Some Walking

Minimal Standing

</td>
<td rowspan="4">

Mental/ Behavioral Health Developmental/Sensory/ADHD Alzheimer/Dementia Concerns?

Ability to:

Understand Instructions

Communicate:

Environmental Reaction:

</td>
</tr>
<tr>
<td>

Hearing:

Some Hearing

Hard of Hearing

</td>
</tr>
<tr>
<td>

Vision:

Some Vision

Minimal Vision

</td>
</tr>
<tr>
<td>

Service Animal:

Type

Name

</td>
</tr>
<tr><td colspan="2">Additional: (Diabetic, Allergies (Latex, Color, Medicines), PTSD, Behavioral Health)</td></tr>
</table>

Very Important People *(To Me!)*

List everyone who lives with the *caree* or visits on a regular basis. Add another sheet if needed.

<table>
<tr><td>
Name:
Relation:
Phone/Cell:
Notes:
</td></tr>
<tr><td>
Name:
Relation:
Phone/Cell:
Notes:
</td></tr>
<tr><td>
Name:
Relation:
Phone/Cell:
Notes:
</td></tr>
<tr><td>
Name:
Relation:
Phone/Cell:
Notes:
</td></tr>
<tr><td>

Service Animal
Name:
Color:
Type:
Note:

</td><td>

Service Animal
Name:
Color:
Type:
Note:

</td></tr>
</table>

Caregiver

Fill this in as if both of you cannot speak and the first responder needs information that is important to your life.

<table>
<tr><td>Personal assistance is needed to:</td></tr>
<tr><td>Caregiver's Name

Phone:
Employer:</td></tr>
<tr><td>My Caregiver is trained to:</td></tr>
<tr><td>If my caregiver is not available, then:</td></tr>
<tr><td>Other:</td></tr>
</table>

Caregiver's Personal FYI Page

-Page Place Holder-

Use this page only for the caregiver to put down any of their own personal medical or disability concerns that first responders might need to know.

Evacuation

Is self-transport/evacuation possible?	Yes No
Assistance needed to get into vehicle	Yes No
Service dog comes with me?	Yes No
Someone will drive caree? Person(s) Identified and Phone Number:	Yes No
Transport Company Used Name & Number: Back-up Plan:	Yes No
Public Transportation What type & Access Point? Back-up Plan:	Yes No
Wheelchair Access Required	Yes No
Power Chair Access Required	Yes No
People & phone numbers who serve as Back-up when there are issues with transportation:	

Home Evacuation Plan

- Page Place Holder -

Outline two different scenarios on how to evacuate the home if there was a fire, gas leak, tornado, or other event such as a fallen tree. Design for basement or second floor evacuations and also plan for main floor blocked standard doorway exits.

An example might be:

2nd Floor: Go down the stairs or outside the window onto the roof.

Main Floor: If front door is blocked use garage door with ramp.

Basement: If basement door is blocked, go out through windows.

You may also want to invite your local fire department to visit your home and have them offer some suggestions or to become aware of the situation.

Third Party Evacuation Plan

– Page Place Holder –

Consider Hotel, Camper, Friend, or Relatives as third party evacuation sites.

Insert Documentation Here
(Examples are: If your caree is in a Nursing Home, Hospice, or attends School etc.)

Medical Biographical Resume

Everyone's medical history is as unique to them as their fingerprint. Use these four pages to create yours. Page one was designed directly with input from paramedics and the medical community, so it would be immediately useful in a life-threatening situation. The sample four pages were created with the needs of the medical community's in mind.

Person's Name / Medical Information as of 5/24/65

Bob Grumby   DOB 12/25/00   Male   Single

0000 Street, City, STATE 30000 Hm: 000.000.0000 Cell: 000.111-0000

Driver's License #   0000000000 Ht. 5'10"   Weight: 000

Social Security: 000.00.0000

Insurance: Insurance Choice, P.O. Box 0000, Albany, KY 00000

Contact info 000.000.0000   Policy/Member ID Z012345678   Group Z0000

Medicare (9/10/00) Member ID: 987654321

IN CASE OF EMERGENCY CONTACT Ginger Spice at 000.999.8888

Highlights:

- Spinal Cord Injury @ T-5 paralyzed from stomach down
- Syringo Pleural Shunt @ T-42x2, partial paralysis in Right Arm
- CRPS
- IYC/Cordis Endovascular Filter: **NO AED Allowed**
- Diabetic II
- Blood Pressure
- **Allergy Alert**
- **Intubation Alert**
- Autonomic Dysreflexia (See page 4) = *[BP + BS + TEMP] x HIGH*
- **Blood Type: O+**
  Transfusions: Jan. 65 - two pints hemoglobin dropped to 5.8 - Island Hospital

IV Administration

Bob's veins are hard to find!!! Suggest using advanced personnel to administer it. Hot cloths placed against arm/hand help. Ultrasound may also help. "IF" and only "if" these don't work… may try the neck.

Note: (found during recent hemorrhoid surgery) Per Hospital on 4/12/64: Need to intubate client due to cranial IX nerve.

MEDICATION SHEET

<u>**Current Prescriptions (taken promptly at 6am & 6pm**</u>

Lyrica	1 capsule	0 mg	1 at morning	Dr. Name
Amitiza	1 capsule	0 mg	1 once a day	Dr. Name
Novolin	R(v-100)		Sliding Scale	Dr. Name
Metoprol Tartrate	1/2 tab	0 mg	1 twice a day	Dr. Name
Humulin	7/0/30	0 units	Every AM & PM	Dr. Name

<u>Self-Medicating</u>

Vitamin w/iron (Multi)	1 tablet		once a day

»Allergies

Betamethasone - side effect of continuous urination
Iron - by IV - had all reactions, breathing, etc.
Lisinoprol - severe - heart attack like symptoms - NO ACE INHIBITORS]
Penicillin - sulfa relationship

Implant (Put in copy of cards here)

Filter: Cordis Endovascular Optease Filter Implant Date
Location: IVC   Dr. Who   Hospital: Medical Center
Address & Phone #
Product: Lot: 0000   Made with Nickel & Titanium   **>>>NO AED** Allowed

Spinal Cord Titanium Rods T2-T10 Cross Bars @T5 and T7
Implant Date
Location: IVC   Dr. Who   Hospital: Medical Center
Address & Phone #
Product: Lot: 0000   Made with Nickel & Titanium   **>>>QUESTION MRI!!!**

<u>MEDICAL CONTACT PAGE</u>

Name	Type	Phone	City	Primary
Dr. Maverick	Family Care/IM	000.000.0000	Hokey Pokey	Yes
Dr. Nevill Chase	Neurologist	000.000.0000	Hokey Pokey	N
Helpful Angels	Nursing Co.	111.111.1111	Nearby	N
Grocery Store	Pharmacy	555.555.5555	Chelsey	N

HOSPITAL ACCOMMODATIONS

In addition to SCI and diabetes II, Jonas has CRPS (Complex Regional Pain Syndrome also known as RSD/Reflex Sympathetic Dystrophy). This means:

RSDSA:Reflex Sympathetic Dystrophy Syndrome Association
http://www.rsds.Org/2/what_is_rsd_crps/index.html
"Complex Regional Pain Syndrome (CRPS), also known as Reflex Sympathetic Dystrophy, is a chronic neurological syndrome characterized by: severe burning pain; pathological changes in bone and skin; excessive sweating; tissue swelling; and extreme sensitivity to touch."

Cleveland Clinic:
http://my.clevelandc1inie.org/anesthesia/publications/archive/complex_pain.aspx

"This is a disease that is characterized by varying degrees of pain and autonomic disturbances that are reflected in changes of the skin, temperature, color and swelling."

Accommodations: (List special equipment needs, medication accommodations, things to make life easier)

Average Daily Schedule
Notes: Medications should be given at 6am/6pm to maintain pain control.
(List a schedule of how medication is administered.)

Bowel/Bladder
Intermittent Cath 4-5 times per day 12 French Soft Bard Complete Kit Cath Bag with Condom Catheter at night only.

HISTORY

If person is medically fragile then list entire medical history presuming you or they can't speak in the situation in as short and as brief a statement as possible: no longer then one page ideally.

Present Symptoms: (List how person is feeling, or any current medical conditions being addressed.) Jonas has been running a temperature and having pain for the past week.

Family History

Mother	Deceased	Age 0	Lung Cancer
Father	Deceased	Age 00	Age

Past Personal History
Has no history of smoking or alcohol intake.

SUPPORTING MEDICAL DOCUMENTATION

<u>SURGICAL / DIAGNOSTIC HISTORY</u>
List hospital visits [Exp.: True Hospital, Smile City, State: 3/5/00 - 3/8/00: Tonsillectomy]

<u>DIAGNOSTIC STUDIES</u>
List all tests, x-rays, MRIs: [Exp.: True Hospital, Smile City, State, 3/5/00]

<u>DOCUMENTATION</u>
Place documentation explaining rare or unknown conditions, diagnosis, disorders.

<u>DAILY SUPPLY LIST</u>

Medical Items
Chucks/Paper Underpads, nitrile gloves *(caregiver is latex allergic),* kitchen garbage bags Bleach Wipes

Wound Care: Saline, Hibiclens, gauze, scissors, Medipore, Mepilex, alcohol wipes
Diabetic Supplies: sugar testing kit, test strips, needles, drinking water

Hardware Needs
Air Mattress & 5 pillows, blanket to protect knees
Transfer Board, Gloves (to move chair and for transferring)

Manual and/or Electric Wheelchair

Batteries for blood sugar testing equipment, blood sugar testing equipment

For Emergency Kit I would add...
Spare battery for power chair, spare tire & kit for manual chair
USB key fob with this packet of data on it, medical bracelet
Gloves to protect hands while turning wheels on chair

*(*** Once this has been created, make extra copies to keep on hand for moment notice emergencies or for the convenience of a new doctor's office!)*

Have you thought of this ?

Do you have Medical Alert Jewelry?   YES   NO

Do you know how to convert the power chair/scooter to manual? Consider putting bright neon dayglo nail polish on the conversion levers for easy identification.

Is there a process to putting together the IV lines? Consider writing down the steps as best you can. Use colors, descriptions and sizes to help identify the steps. Write steps in terms of in positive/negative consequences where appropriate.

What size batteries do the hearing aids or walking canes take? Note date and how often they should be replaced.

What is the back-up plan for not having to assistive technology when it is not available? Are there spare batteries? If so, where? What happens if the technology is not available? How else can that daily life skill be accommodated?

Are there tubes and bandages that need to be replaced multiple times and on multiple days? Do you have some set aside in your To-Go kit?

If there's a piece of equipment that there is only one of, what is the alternative back-up plan if it gets destroyed in a disaster or left behind when quickly evacuating? (Such as a transfer board, crutches, or seizure helmet.)

Is a device or object needed to keep the caree calm? Yes No, if yes, what is it? What is its purpose?

Internal Body Equipment

Insert Information for Internal Body Equipment (Plastic/Metal Parts/Platinum) which can include, but is not limited to:

Vena Cava Catheters	Hip Replacements
Shunts	Pace Makers
Spinal Cord Injury Rods	Defibrillators
Catheters	

If the hospital issued you an identification card (with Model/Serial/Date) for your records and/or to use at the airport; tape and/or Xerox copy of it to this page. *(This is also good knowledge for recalls and MRI magnetism concerns!)*

Technology:

Type of Equipment:

Model Numbers:

Company Purchased from:

Phone:

Technology:

Type of Equipment:

Model Numbers:

Company Purchased from:

Phone:

External Body Equipment

Provide or attach any technology identification data on this page too!

Limb Prosthesis Body Location:	Type:
Limb Guard Body Location:	Type:
Orthotics Body Location	Type:
(Select) **Crutches / Walker / Cane** Used for:	

Hearing Aid	Right	Left
Glass Eye	Right	Left
Other		

Technology:

Type of Equipment:

Model Numbers:

Company Purchased from:

Phone:

Insert information for sensory concerns associated with making transport and evaluation as comfortable as possible for your caree. For example, if your caree is sensitive to sound you may consider having headphones listed as an accommodation.

Tactile (Touch, Air Movement from Fans, etc.)
Hearing (Loud, Multiple, Sharp, Lights, Crowds)
Visual (Light, Color)
Smell (Perfume, Cleaning Chemical, Smoke)
Air Quality (Temperature, Humidity, Barometric)

Unusual or Rare Diagnosis or Condition

-Page Place Holder-

Consider adding brochures or flyers or even your own letter.

Insert Description of Unusual or Rare Diagnosis or Condition Definition Here

Example:

- Epilepsy

- Pulmonary Arterial Hypertension

- Complex Regional Pain Disorder

- Syringomyelia

- P.A.N.D.A.S. Pediatric Autoimmune Neuropsychiatric Disorder Association with Streptococcal infection.

Infection Control

Contact your local health department for more education on this. This is important to know regardless of the location and may end up being especially handy knowledge in an emergency shelter situation.

Hand-washing
- Wash hands thoroughly before and after every time you work with your caree for 20 seconds. Including when having contact with:
  * Any bodily fluids
  * Food preparation and handling
  * Any medical equipment or environment

National Caregivers Library:
Infection Control (c) 1999-2013 Family Care America, Inc. 11414

http://www.caregiverslibrary.org/caregivers-resources/grp-home-care/infection-control-article.aspx

Glove Protection
Using latex/vinyl/nitrile gloves can help both you and your caree from catching bacteria that could be seriously harmful.

- Do not use gloves more than once as it can reintroduce bacteria.
- Do not use gloves that are damaged or imperfect in any manner.
- Sometimes they may be covered under insurance policies.

National Caregivers Library:
Wearing Gloves (c) 1999-2013 Family Care America, Inc. 11414

http://www.caregiverslibrary.org/caregivers-resources/grp-diseases/hsgrp-hiv-aids/wearing-gloves-article.aspx

Clean Work Environment
- Set up a clean work area.
- Have plenty of supplies.
- Be careful not to allow medical supplies to be touched by hands or placed directly onto tables unless they are covered properly.
- Have plenty of garbage bags and bleach wipes to clean up with afterwards.
- Place needles and other used medical items in appropriate containers.

Long Distance Contacts Checklist

Enter in the name and contact for each or insert a page of your own. Make sure to include the state so time zone issues can be considered.

Nearby Family
Neighbors
Friends
Religious Community
Utilities
Landscaper
Housekeeper
Social Groups
Social Worker
Nearby Community Specific Contacts

Hospice Details

-Page Place Holder-

Insert/attach any special instructions, conditions or events that Caregivers and First Responders should be aware of.

Contacts are important too:

Organization/City	Contact Name/ Title	Phone/ Email
Hospice Organization		
Social Worker		
Power of Attorney		
Personal Advocate		
Family		

Copy of Will/Medical Directives

-Page Place Holder-

This could also be a place for the Power of Attorney and other important documents. If there's a concern about placing them in the book, then put down the name and contact number of who has them or would know where to find them.

Disaster Preparedness

1. Prepare Home and an Away To-Go kit for you and your caree to be able to take care of yourselves. (See resources on back for suggestions for kit items.)
2. Make sure you are trained on your caree's equipment intimately, know how to break it down and put it back together again.
3. Create a complete detailed medical document of your caree which includes their diagnoses(is), medicine, hardware/software needs, and personal assistance that they would need on a daily basis. //Don't forget to create a printout (or USB key / or plastic refrigerator pocket) of your own medications too!
4. Get a medic alert bracelet with the text notating that you are a caregiver for someone who has *(fill in the blank)*.
5. Make your plans to be flexible for the many types of disaster or challenges that can occur.
6. For every aspect of the emergency plan you create for your caree, create two more: one as an alternative and the other when the first two fail.
7. Identify at least 3 other people (trained) to fill the caregiving role in case you are on the other side of town or medically incapacitated when a disaster occurs.
8. Understand that when you are with your caree you are the *'first'* responder on the scene when a disaster occurs.
9. Reach out to your local Fire Department, Emergency Management Office and/or Health Department and ask them to connect you with emergency planning resources/ tools that would be catered to the specifics of your caree's situation.
10. Make sure the nursing home, assisted living facility, personal care home, therapy, caregiving assistance entities that you work with also have emergency preparedness planning that covers your caree...and if not make sure one is created to your liking.
11. Take a CPR or Certified Caregiving Course.
12. Take a community CERT (Community Emergency Response Team) course. This does not mean that you have to sign up and help them necessarily; but it's a great place to learn how to put out small house fires, address utility problems, and very basic disaster protection. (See for more information: http://www.fema.gov/community-emergency-response-teams)
13. Work with your caree to make sure they know what to do and understand the plan's importance. If they don't have the capacity to participate then write this aspect into your plans.
14. Don't forget to make plans for yourself, loved ones and pets as it will be difficult for the caree if they have to worry about you too!

Caregiver Organization Emergency Preparedness Resources

US DHHS AOA (Administration on Aging)
National Family Caregiver Support Program

Emergency Readiness for Older Adults and Caregivers

http ://www.aoa. gov/AoAJPrograms/HCLTC/Caregiver/docs/

Just_in_Case030706_links.pdf

CDC (Centers for Disease Control)
Emergency Preparedness for Older Adults

Personal Preparedness for Older Adults and their Caregivers

http://www.cdc.gov/aging/emergency/preparedness.htm

National Center on Caregiving
Emergency Preparedness on Caregiving

https://caregiver.org/emergency-preparedness-checklist-caregivers

US DHHS ASPR (Assistant Secretary for Preparedness and Response)
Public Health Emergency

Disaster Preparedness for Family Caregivers Webinar (Dated 4/16/14)
http://www.phe.gov/preparedness/planning/abc/pages/caregiver-webinar.aspx

Rosalynn Carter Institute for Caregiving
CARE-NET (Caregivers Network) Volunteer Coalition of caregiver support
organizations across a broad array of illnesses and disabilities. http
://www.rosalynncarter. org/

NextAvenue
Why Caregivers Need to Plan for the Worst

Whether your loved ones live alone or in a nursing home, be ready to help them
in case of disaster, by Sherri Snelling, 4/22/13

http://www.nextavenue.org/article/2012-07/why-caregivers-need-plan-worst

NATIONAL COUNCIL ON INDEPENDENT LIVING
Select the statewide office or the local office needed.
http://www.NCIL.org

REGIONAL INDEPENDENT LIVING CENTER
(Go the following link then, select the state, then the region:
http://www.ILRU.org/projects/cil-net/cil-center-and-association-directory.)

YOUR PERSONAL COMMUNITY SUPPORT ORGANIZATION

OTHER

Local First Responder Resources

These organizations really would like to answer your questions and offer additional resources to help complete this workbook!

(Enter Organization, Contact Name, Number and Social Media Connections)

POLICE DEPARTMENT

FIRE DEPARTMENT

COMMUNITY/LOCAL EMERGENCY PREPAREDNESS COALITION

Make sure you have a fire/CO2 alarm. If not, reach out to your local fire department as most have programs to help with that. While you are there, get connected to their community alert notification program.

CITY EMA OFFICE

COUNTY EMA OFFICE

COUNTY HEALTH DEPARTMENT

(Edit with your own state.)

STATE EMA OFFICE

STATE ADA OFFICE

STATE HEALTH DEPARTMENT

READY.Gov
Preparing Makes Sense for People with Disabilities and Special Needs
http://www.ready.gov/document/preparing-makes-sense-people-disabilities-and-special-needs

FEDERAL EMERGENCY MANAGEMENT AGENCY (FEMA)
U.S. Department of Homeland Security
500 C Street Southwest
Washington, D.C. 20472

Disaster Assistance: 800.621.3362 / TTY 800.462.7585

Ph: 202.646.2500

www.fema.gov

FB: FEMA

Twitter: FEMA

YouTube: FEMA

CENTERS FOR DISEASE CONTROL (CDC) AND PREVENTION
1600 Clifton Road
Atlanta, GA 30329-4027

Ph: 800.CDC-INFO (800.232.4636)
www.cdc.gov (and RSS feed)

FB: CDC
Twitter: CDCgov

Miscellaneous Helpful Notes

Home Health Care Company: Find out if they have an Emergency Preparedness plan for your caree while in their care, and if not encourage them to do so.

Medication: To have spare medication on hand, ask the doctor if he will write a script for an extra week's worth. It might be necessary to check with the insurance company in which some will issue an extra month's worth. Use this scenario for catheters, tubing and other supplies that be acquired on a regular basis.

Comfort Items: Some children and adults rely on technology, stuffed animals or other items to comfort and calm them down. Consider adding that to this workbook with a description of how it calms them and the importance of it.

Meet-up Plan: If you get separated have a designated hospital, friend's home or other location to meet-up at in addition to a phone number to reach each other.

Nationwide Databases: Take advantage of this technology to list the medications with a nationwide pharmacy and to access funds regardless of the location.

Phone Contact Tree: Rather than creating a list of only one contact, think in terms of multiples. Thus, three emergency family contacts, three home health agency contacts, three school contacts, and so on. File a copy with a local family member (or someone you trust), a regional or state out of town contact and with the primary physician.

Social Media: Since I initially wrote this book, both emergency management and consumers have made it an invaluable resource in a disaster. There are good and bad sides to this. Good for getting information quickly and if you find the right site you can get most of the needed information in one place. Bad, if you are not careful to make sure that the site is sharing reliable and confirmable information. Do not post your address publicly for your safety. If you are in a dire situation and cannot reach first responders through your community tread carefully with who you share your information with.

Notes

This page is for you to add in anything else that might not be in this document yet important to the well-being of both the caree and caregiver in an emergency.

Technology Tools for Emergency Preparedness

The importance of a backup plan cannot be reiterated enough. Using this workbook is a great way to begin your emergency preparedness planning. In the event that the guide is misplaced or damaged during the emergency, having an electronic way to easily access your information is a good backup plan.

Located at https://mindlight.io/ you can get access to a free web application, a link to a free iPhone application, or a link to a free Android application. Each of these will take you to an app made for family caregivers by family caregivers to connect, coordinate, and communication.

You can use the app to invite team members into your emergency preparedness team, store important documents like a copy of this guide, store and share important contacts and locations that are important in an emergency, create a task list to share with others on what you need help with, and use the chat functionality to keep everyone on the team up to date with the status of the emergency.

This app can be used outside of emergency planning as well. If you are a parent of a special child, a caregiver for someone with disabilities or the elderly, or just have a complex care situation – this app is designed to keep everyone in your care team connected, coordinated, and facilitates communication.

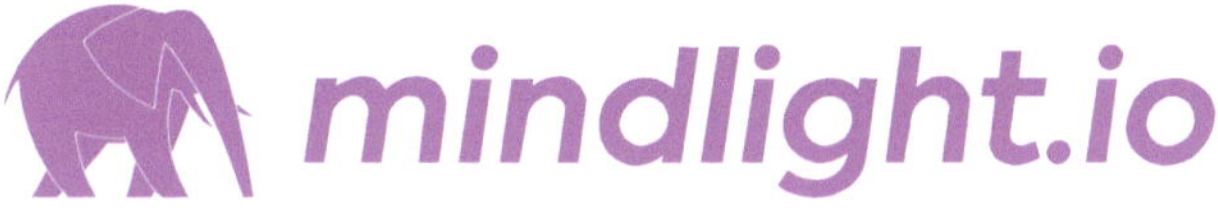

Congratulations!

This is now the plan that speaks for the both the caregiver and caree. It was not that hard, yet it also gave you time to really think about 'what if'. To make this plan even better and stronger, consider working on this workbook on a regular basis (*...if you haven't completed it yet!*) and with anyone who works in the first responding community to learn what resources they have that would help you to recover from an emergency quickly. Each time this book has new data entered makes your plan more helpful when needed in an emergency. Do not be afraid to add extra pages or move the pages around. ***This is your book!*** Do whatever it takes to make this able to speak for you...when you or someone you trust cannot speak.

It was my pleasure to create this tool as means to help keep you and all those you care about around you safe. Much of these questions are things you may have never thought about until now. But having put this booklet together you are now empowered to be safer in a disaster and not solely dependent on those who may not know how to help you.

Now make paper copies, USB key copies and distribute them to people who you trust to speak on your behalf following your wishes. Also, please don't hesitate to let me know how this helped you or offer any additional thoughts that you think might be added to this to help others.

Prepare to be Ready!

Laura George
Emergency Management Disability Liaison
LauraGeorgeEMDL@gmail.com

About the Author

Laura George has spent over 12 years working with the emergency management, disability, elderly, caregiving, and other communities to encourage positive collaboration on pre/during/post disaster planning. Her work in this field was prompted when she had to choose between her newly paralyzed spouse, her unborn child and an impending hurricane.

Even though she has a Bachelor of Science from Nova Southeastern University, her actual education came from her experiences as a caregiver for her husband and later for her daughter. Having received multiple certifications, she feels her best education came from her experiences participating in many committees and gathering personal stories shared with her over the years. Several of these stories come from assisting in disasters such as Sandy, Snowmageddon, Florence and now Michael.

Laura has written for a wide variety of publications including Exceptional Magazine, Georgia Council on Developmental Disabilities, Abilities Expo, and Florida Spinal Cord Injury Resource Center. Currently she sits on local, state and national committees and manages three social media preparedness sites which offer preparedness tips and community alert notifications.

She has received many awards and accolades for her uncharted and compassionate work. Most notable are the 2011 Caregiver of the Year Award for the Atlanta Region ARC - Rosalynn Carter Institute and the 2011 HomeWatch Caregivers Northeast Atlanta Region. Prior to that she shared with her husband in receiving the 2008 South Florida Center for Independent Living: Advocates of the Year Award; *"for their commitment and hard work to enhance services for People with Disabilities."*

It is Laura's continued hope that awareness, education and collaborative inclusion of the disabled, elderly and other communities will evolve to meaningful and positive emergency management design.

She would love to hear from you at:
Facebook: https://www.facebook.com/groups/LauraGeorgeEMDL/

Email: LauraGeorgeEMDL@gmail.com